Positive Thinking

By

Sagittarius Partey

TO MY MOTHER, MOSIBURAT BASHORUN

My Orisa.

PREFACE

It's a common issue that affects people of all ages and backgrounds. While everyone experiences negative thoughts from time to time, it's important to recognize when they become a persistent pattern that impacts our daily lives.

In this book, I've drawn on my experience as well as the latest research in psychology to offer practical strategies for overcoming negative thoughts and emotions. Whether you're struggling with anxiety, depression, or simply feeling stuck in a negative mindset, this book is designed to help you develop a more positive outlook on life.

The strategies outlined in this book aren't a quick fix or a magic cure. It takes time and effort to cultivate a positive mindset, but the benefits are well worth it. By practicing these techniques and exercises, you can transform your thinking patterns and improve your mental wellbeing.

I hope this book will serve as a valuable resource for anyone seeking to cultivate positivity and overcome negative thinking. Remember, change is possible, and small steps can make a big difference in improving your overall quality of life.

Sagittarius Partey

FOREWORD

In today's fast-paced and often stressful world, it's easy to get bogged down by negative thoughts and emotions. From personal setbacks to global crises, it can be all too easy to feel discouraged, hopeless, and overwhelmed.

But as the author of this book, "The Power of Positive Thinking," reminds us, there is another way. By cultivating a positive mindset, we can overcome obstacles, build resilience, and achieve our goals. Drawing on the latest research in psychology, neuroscience, and self-help, this book offers practical strategies for developing a positive outlook and creating a more fulfilling life.

With its clear and engaging writing style, this book is a valuable resource for anyone who wants to harness the power of positive thinking. Whether you're struggling with stress, anxiety, or self-doubt, or simply looking to improve your overall well-being, the insights and techniques in this book can help you to cultivate a more positive and optimistic mindset.

So, whether you're a seasoned self-help reader or just starting out on your personal growth journey, I highly recommend this book. It's a powerful reminder that, no matter what challenges we face, we always have the power to choose our mindset and create a brighter future for ourselves and those around us.

Best wishes,

Sagittarius Partey

INTRODUCTION

Positive thinking is a mental attitude that involves focusing on the positive aspects of life and the potential for good outcomes. It involves cultivating optimism, gratitude, and a can-do attitude, and seeing setbacks as temporary and surmountable. Positive thinking has been shown to have many benefits, including improved mental health, greater resilience, and better physical health.

Positive thinking is a complex and multifaceted field that encompasses a range of concepts and findings related to the impact of our thoughts and emotions on our brains and overall well-being. By understanding these concepts and engaging in practices that promote positive thinking, individuals can enhance their mental health and well-being, and build greater resilience and fulfillment in their lives.

Overall, a positive mindset can have a significant impact on all aspects of an individual's life, promoting greater health, happiness, and success.

HOW NEGATIVE THINKING AFFECTS OUR MENTAL HEALTH

Negative thinking can have a profound effect on our mental health. When we consistently have negative thoughts, it can lead to feelings of anxiety, depression, and low self-esteem. Here are some ways in which negative thinking can affect our mental health:

1. ***Increases anxiety***: *Negative thinking patterns can lead to increased anxiety and worry. When we consistently have negative thoughts, we tend to focus on worst-case scenarios and become overly concerned about the future. This can lead to feelings of anxiety and stress.*

2. ***Leads to depression***: *Negative thinking can also lead to depression. When we constantly focus on negative events or aspects of our lives, it can lead to feelings of hopelessness, helplessness, and sadness. This can then lead to depression.*

3. ***Low self-esteem***: *Negative thinking can also contribute to low self-esteem. When we consistently have negative thoughts about ourselves, our abilities, or our appearance, it can lead to feelings of inadequacy and low self-worth.*

4. ***Impacts relationships***: *Negative thinking can also impact our relationships. When we constantly focus on negative aspects of our partners or friends, it can lead to conflict and distance in our relationships.*

5. ***Reduced motivation***: *Negative thinking can make it difficult to feel motivated or to take action, as individuals may feel that their efforts are futile or that they will fail.*

6. ***Difficulty coping with stress***: *Negative thinking can make it difficult to cope with stressful situations, as individuals may feel overwhelmed and unable to handle the demands of the situation.*

Overall, negative thinking can have a significant impact on our mental health. It's important to be aware of our thought patterns and try to reframe negative thoughts into more positive ones. This can help to improve our mood, reduce anxiety, and improve our overall mental health.

Sagittarius Partey

TABLE OF CONTENT

CHAPTER 1

THE SCIENCE OF POSITIVE THINKING

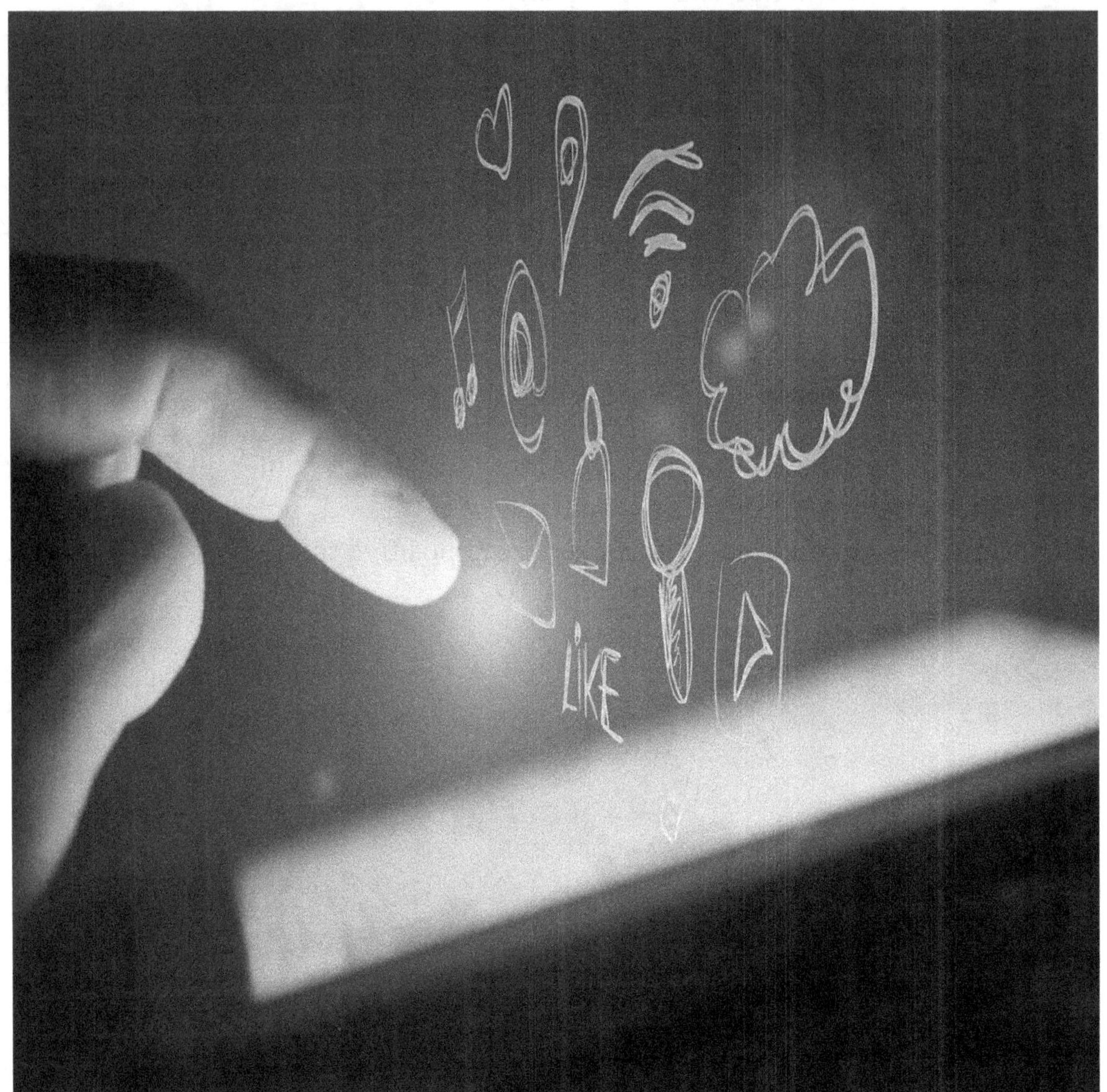

Research has shown that positive thinking can have a significant impact on the brain. Neuroplasticity, the brain's ability to change and adapt in response to experience, is a key factor in this. Positive thinking has been shown to increase activity in the prefrontal cortex, which is associated with decision-making, planning, and problem-solving. Gratitude and

mindfulness have also been shown to have positive effects on the brain, including

reducing stress and anxiety.

Positive thinking has been studied extensively in the field of psychology, and there

is evidence to suggest that it can have a significant impact on our brains and

overall well-being. Here are some of the key findings from research on the science

of positive thinking:

Here are some additional findings and concepts related to the science of positive

thinking:

1. **The positivity ratio**: The positivity ratio is a concept that refers to the
   balance between positive and negative emotions in our lives. Research
   suggests that a ratio of three positive emotions to one negative emotion is
   optimal for promoting mental health and well-being.

2. **The broaden-and-build theory**: The broaden-and-build theory suggests
   that positive emotions, such as joy and contentment, can broaden our
   perspectives and cognitive abilities, allowing us to think more creatively and
   flexibly. This, in turn, can lead to a range of benefits, including increased
   resilience and enhanced social connections.

3. **The self-fulfilling prophecy**: The self-fulfilling prophecy is a concept that refers to the idea that our beliefs about ourselves and the world can shape our experiences and outcomes. For example, if we believe that we are capable of achieving our goals, we are more likely to take action and succeed, whereas if we believe that we are destined to fail, we are more likely to give up and not even try.

4. **The power of positive affirmations**: Positive affirmations are statements that we repeat to ourselves in order to promote positive thinking and self-belief. Research suggests that positive affirmations can have a significant impact on our self-perception and self-esteem, as well as our ability to cope with stress and adversity.

HOW POSITIVE THINKING AFFECTS THE BRAIN

When we think positively, our brains release neurotransmitters such as dopamine and serotonin, which promote feelings of pleasure and well-being. This can lead to a more positive outlook on life and greater resilience in the face of stress and adversity

Positive thinking can have a significant impact on the brain, both in the short term and the long term. Here are some ways that positive thinking can affect the brain:

1. **Reducing stress**: Positive thinking can help reduce stress levels, which can have a positive impact on the brain. When we're stressed, our body produces cortisol, a hormone that can have negative effects on the brain, such as impairing memory and increasing the risk of depression. By reducing stress levels through positive thinking, we can protect our brain from these negative effects.

2. **Increasing resilience**: Positive thinking can also help increase our resilience, which is our ability to bounce back from difficult situations. By focusing on the positive aspects of a situation, we can develop a more

optimistic outlook and a greater sense of control, which can help us cope with challenges more effectively.

3. **Boosting mood**: When we think positively, we release feel-good chemicals in our brain, such as dopamine and serotonin. These chemicals can improve our mood, increase our sense of well-being, and even reduce pain.

4. **Improving cognitive function**: Positive thinking can also improve cognitive function, such as memory, attention, and decision-making. This is because positive thoughts help to activate the prefrontal cortex, which is the part of the brain responsible for these functions.

Overall, positive thinking can have a powerful impact on the brain, helping to reduce stress, increase resilience, boost mood, and improve cognitive function.

Here are some additional ways that positive thinking can affect the brain:

5. **Enhancing creativity**: When we think positively, we're more likely to approach problems and challenges with a flexible and open-minded mindset. This can help to enhance our creativity and innovation, as we're more willing to consider new ideas and approaches.

6. **Strengthening relationships**: Positive thinking can also have a positive impact on our social connections and relationships. When we have a positive outlook, we're more likely to be kind, empathetic, and supportive towards

others, which can strengthen our connections and improve our social well-being.

7. **Boosting physical health**: In addition to its effects on the brain, positive thinking can also have a positive impact on our physical health. Studies have shown that people with a positive outlook are more likely to engage in healthy behaviors, such as exercise and healthy eating, and have lower rates of chronic diseases such as heart disease and diabetes.

8. **Increasing longevity**: Finally, positive thinking may even increase our longevity. Research has shown that people with a positive outlook on life tend to live longer and have a lower risk of premature death, possibly due to the protective effects of positive emotions on the body and mind.

9. **Improved mental health**: Positive thinking can help reduce symptoms of anxiety and depression, as well as increase overall life satisfaction and happiness.

10. **Greater resilience**: A positive mindset helps individuals cope with stress and adversity more effectively, bouncing back from setbacks more easily and quickly.

11. **Better physical health**: Studies have shown that positive thinking is associated with improved immune system function, lower blood pressure, and reduced risk of chronic diseases such as heart disease and diabetes.

12. **Enhanced relationships**: Positive individuals tend to attract and maintain positive relationships, leading to greater social support and a more fulfilling social life.

13. **Improved productivity**: A positive mindset can lead to increased motivation, creativity, and productivity, as individuals are more likely to approach tasks with a can-do attitude and a sense of optimism.

In summary, positive thinking can affect the brain in numerous ways, from reducing stress and increasing resilience to boosting mood, improving cognitive function, enhancing creativity, strengthening relationships, promoting physical health, and even increasing longevity

Overall, the science of positive thinking suggests that our thoughts and emotions have a powerful impact on our brains and overall well-being. By cultivating a positive mindset and engaging in practices that promote positive thinking, individuals can enhance their mental health and build greater resilience in the face of stress and adversity.

THE POWER OF NEUROPLASTICITY

The brain has the ability to change and adapt in response to experiences and environmental factors, a process known as neuroplasticity. Research suggests that positive thinking can promote neuroplasticity, allowing the brain to create new neural pathways and strengthen existing ones.

THE ROLE OF GRATITUDE AND MINDFULNESS

Research has shown that practices such as gratitude journaling and mindfulness meditation can have a significant impact on mental health and well-being. These practices can help promote positive thinking by encouraging individuals to focus on the present moment and cultivate a sense of gratitude for the positive aspects of their lives.

CHAPTER 2

IDENTIFYING NEGATIVE THOUGHT PATTERNS

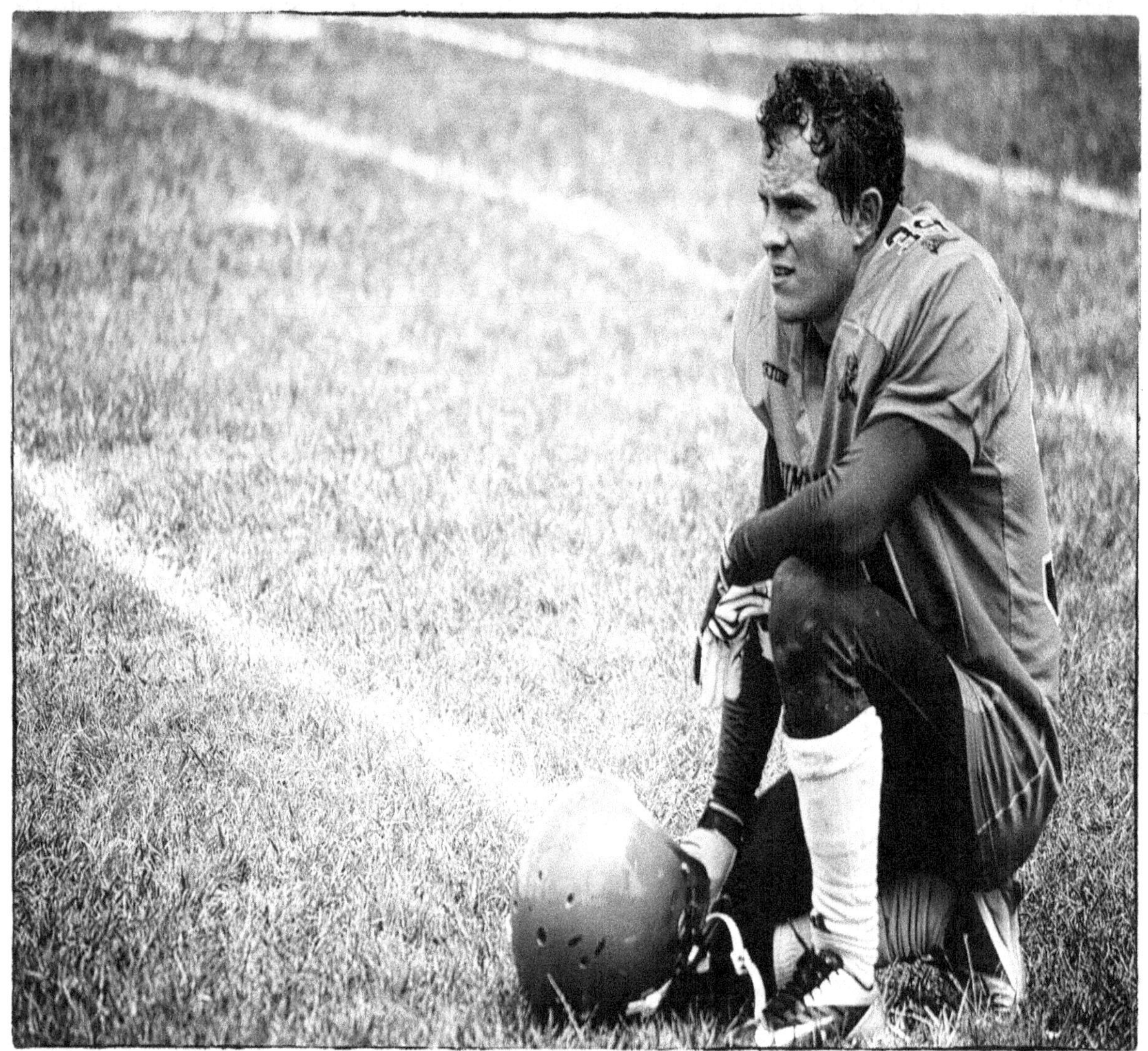

Negative thinking can have a detrimental effect on mental health, and it is important to recognize and challenge negative thought patterns. Common negative thought patterns include black-and-white thinking, catastrophizing, and personalization. Negative self-talk can also be damaging, as it can lead to low self-esteem and self-doubt. Tools such as cognitive-behavioral therapy can help individuals recognize and challenge negative thoughts.

COMMON NEGATIVE THOUGHT PATTERNS

1. **All-or-Nothing Thinking**: This is a pattern of negative thinking where you view situations in terms of extremes, such as "good or bad," "right or wrong," "success or failure," etc.

2. **Overgeneralization**: This is a pattern of negative thinking where you draw broad conclusions based on limited evidence, often leading to negative self-talk and self-doubt.

3. **Mental Filtering**: This is a pattern of negative thinking where you selectively focus on negative aspects of a situation and filter out the positive aspects.

4. **Mind Reading**: This is a pattern of negative thinking where you assume you know what other people are thinking or feeling, often leading to negative assumptions and misunderstandings

5. **Magnification and Minimization**: This is a pattern of negative thinking where you exaggerate the negative aspects of a situation and minimize the positive aspects, often leading to feelings of anxiety and depression.

6. **Catastrophizing**: This is a pattern of negative thinking where you imagine the worst-case scenario, often leading to feelings of fear, helplessness, and

hopelessness.

7. **Emotional Reasoning**: This is a pattern of negative thinking where you believe your emotions are a reflection of reality, often leading to irrational thoughts and behaviors.

8. **Personalization**: This is a pattern of negative thinking where you take things personally and assume responsibility for things that are not your fault.

9. **Should Statements**: This is a pattern of negative thinking where you use words like "should," "must," or "ought to" to impose unrealistic expectations on yourself and others, often leading to feelings of guilt and shame.

10. **Self-Blame**: This is a pattern of negative thinking where you blame yourself for things that are not entirely your fault, often leading to feelings of low self-esteem and self-doubt.

THE IMPACT OF NEGATIVE SELF-TALK

1. **Increased Stress**: Negative self-talk can cause increased stress levels, which can lead to physical and mental health problems.

2. **Decreased Self-Confidence**: Negative self-talk can erode self-confidence and self-esteem, leading to a negative cycle of self-doubt and self-criticism.

3. **Increased Anxiety and Depression**: Negative self-talk can contribute to feelings of anxiety and depression, which can be debilitating and affect daily life.

4. **Reduced Motivation**: Negative self-talk can sap motivation and lead to a lack of enthusiasm for activities, projects, and goals.

5. **Limited Creativity**: Negative self-talk can limit creativity and prevent individuals from exploring new ideas and solutions to problems.

6. **Strained Relationships**: Negative self-talk can lead to strained relationships with others, as it can cause individuals to feel insecure, defensive, or overly critical.

7. **Limited Creativity**: Negative self-talk can limit creativity and prevent individuals from exploring new ideas and solutions to problems.

8. **Strained Relationships**: Negative self-talk can lead to strained relationships with others, as it can cause individuals to feel insecure, defensive, or overly critical.

9.**Reduced Resilience**: Negative self-talk can reduce resilience and prevent individuals from bouncing back from setbacks and challenges.

10. **Limited Growth**: Negative self-talk can limit personal growth and prevent individuals from reaching their full potential.

TOOLS FOR RECOGNIZING AND CHALLENGING NEGATIVE THOUGHTS

1. **Mindfulness**: Mindfulness involves paying attention to the present moment without judgment. This can help you recognize negative thoughts as they arise and prevent them from taking over.

2. **Cognitive Restructuring**: This involves challenging negative thoughts by examining evidence for and against them and replacing them with more positive, realistic thoughts.

3. **Thought Stopping**: This involves recognizing negative thoughts as they arise and stopping them in their tracks by saying "stop" or another word or phrase that helps you shift your focus.

4. **Journaling**: Writing down negative thoughts can help you recognize patterns and develop strategies for challenging them.

5. **Gratitude**: Practicing gratitude can help shift your focus away from negative thoughts and help you see the positive aspects of your life.

6. **Positive Self-Talk**: Using positive self-talk can help counteract negative thoughts and reinforce positive beliefs about yourself.

7. **Mind-Body Techniques**: Techniques such as deep breathing, yoga, and meditation can help you reduce stress and anxiety and develop a more positive outlook.

8. **Social Support**: Seeking support from friends, family, or a therapist can help

you gain perspective and challenge negative thoughts.

9. **Goal Setting**: Setting achievable goals and focusing on accomplishments can help boost self-esteem and counteract negative thinking.

10. **Self-Care**: Taking care of your physical, emotional, and mental health can help you feel more positive and resilient in the face of negative thoughts and emotions.

CHAPTER 3

REPLACING NEGATIVE THOUGHTS WITH POSITIVE ONES

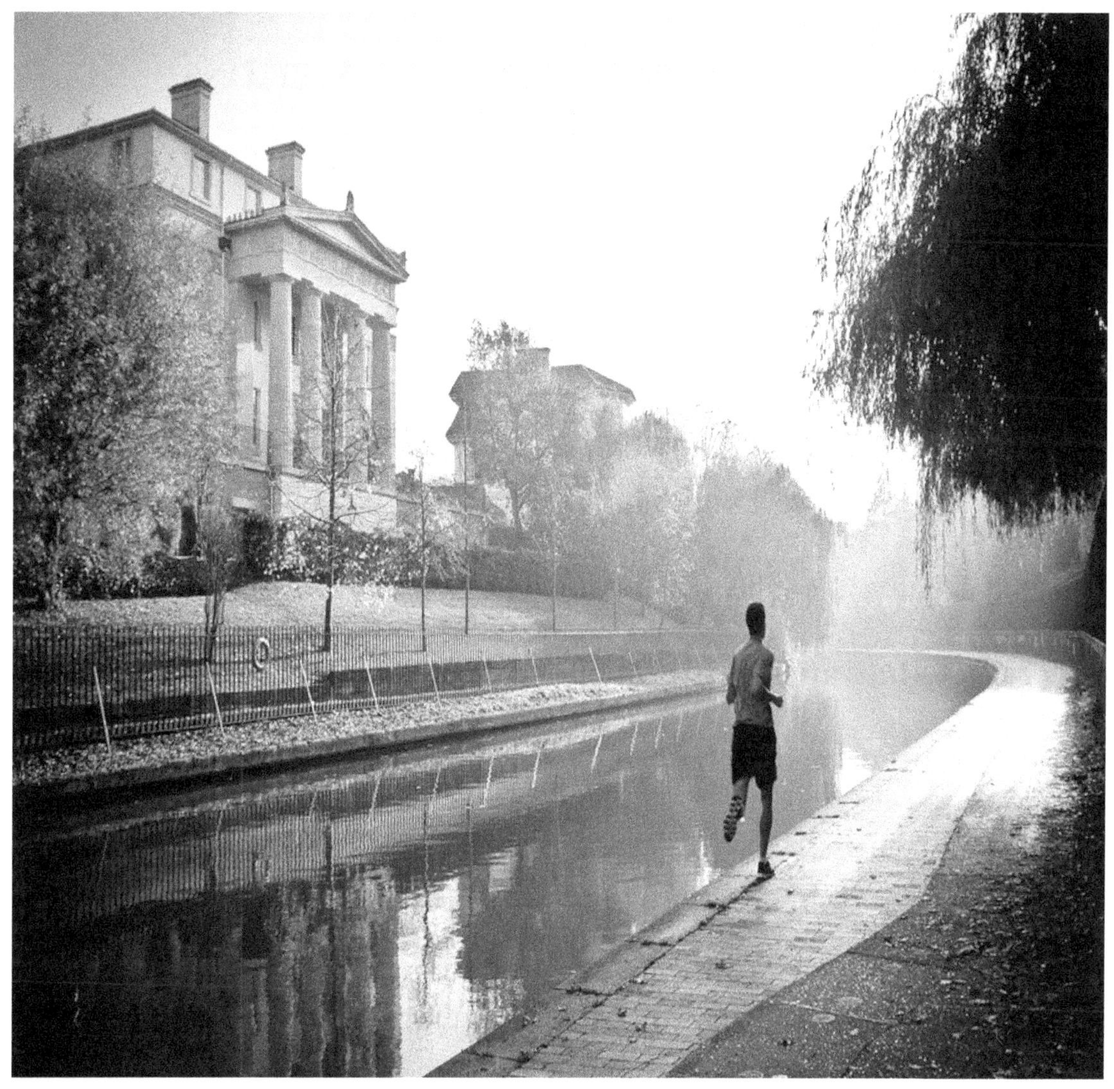

There are many techniques for replacing negative thoughts with positive ones. Affirmations, which involve repeating positive statements to oneself, can be a powerful tool for promoting positive thinking. Reframing negative situations involves looking for the positive aspects of a situation and focusing on them. Visualization techniques involve imagining positive outcomes and can help individuals feel more confident and motivated.

THE POWER OF AFFIRMATIONS

1. **Boosts Self-Confidence**: Affirmations can boost self-confidence by promoting positive self-talk and self-beliefs.

2. **Reduces Stress**: Positive affirmations can reduce stress by helping to calm the mind and promote a more positive outlook.

3. **Encourages Positive Thinking**: Affirmations encourage positive thinking by replacing negative thoughts with positive ones.

4. **Increases Motivation**: Affirmations can increase motivation by promoting positive self-beliefs and encouraging individuals to take action towards their goals.

5. **Enhances Self-Esteem**: Affirmations can enhance self-esteem by promoting positive self-beliefs and self-worth.

6. **Improves Relationships**: Affirmations can improve relationships by promoting positive communication and reinforcing positive beliefs about oneself and others.

7. **Boosts Resilience**: Affirmations can boost resilience by promoting positive self-beliefs and helping individuals bounce back from setbacks and challenges.

8. **Increases Creativity**: Affirmations can increase creativity by promoting positive self-beliefs and encouraging individuals to explore new ideas and solutions.

9. **Improves Physical Health**: Affirmations can improve physical health by reducing stress and promoting a positive outlook, which can lead to improved immune function and overall health.

10. **Promotes Personal Growth**: Affirmations can promote personal growth by encouraging individuals to challenge limiting beliefs and develop a more positive and empowered self-image.

REFRAMING NEGATIVE SITUATIONS

1. **Look for Evidence**: Examine the evidence for and against the negative thought and try to come up with a more balanced perspective.

2. **Reframe the Thought**: Turn a negative thought into a positive one by finding an alternative, more positive way of looking at the situation.

3. **Practice Gratitude**: Focus on the positive aspects of your life and the things you are grateful for to counteract negative thoughts.

4. **Use Humor**: Sometimes using humor to reframe negative thoughts can help lighten the mood and put things into perspective.

5. **Challenge Assumptions**: Question any assumptions or beliefs that underlie negative thoughts to see if they are truly accurate or helpful.

6. **Shift Your Focus**: Redirect your attention to something positive or engaging to distract yourself from negative thoughts.

7. **Use Affirmations**: Use positive affirmations to counteract negative self-talk and promote more positive beliefs about yourself.

8. **Practice Mindfulness**: Observe your negative thoughts without judgment and focus on the present moment to reduce their impact.

9. **Seek Support**: Talk to a trusted friend or therapist to gain perspective and support in reframing negative thoughts.

10. **Take Action**: Sometimes taking action towards a goal or addressing a problem

can help reframe negative thoughts by empowering you to take control of the

situation.

USING VISUALIZATION TECHNIQUES

1. **Create a Vision Board**: Collect images and quotes that represent your goals and aspirations and create a collage or visual representation of them to keep them in mind.

2. **Guided Imagery**: Listen to guided meditations or visualizations that help you imagine positive outcomes and experiences.

3. **Mental Rehearsal**: Practice visualizing yourself succeeding in a particular task or activity, such as giving a presentation or performing in a competition.

4. **Positive Self-Talk**: Use positive affirmations and self-talk to reinforce positive beliefs and help you visualize success.

5. **Create a Mental Sanctuary**: Visualize a peaceful and calming place, such as a beach or forest, and imagine yourself relaxing and letting go of stress.

6. **Visualize Your Ideal Day**: Imagine your ideal day, from the moment you wake up to the activities you enjoy and the people you interact with.

7. **Future Self Visualization**: Imagine yourself in the future, having achieved your goals and living the life you desire.

8. **Use Imagery to Overcome Obstacles**: Visualize yourself overcoming challenges and obstacles by using creative problem-solving and perseverance.

9. **Positive Outcome Visualization**: Visualize a positive outcome to a difficult situation, such as a successful job interview or resolving a conflict with a loved

one.

10. **Practice Mindful Visualization**: Practice visualization techniques with mindful awareness and focus, being fully present in the moment and using all of your senses to enhance the experience.

CHAPTER 4

BUILDING A POSITIVE MINDSET

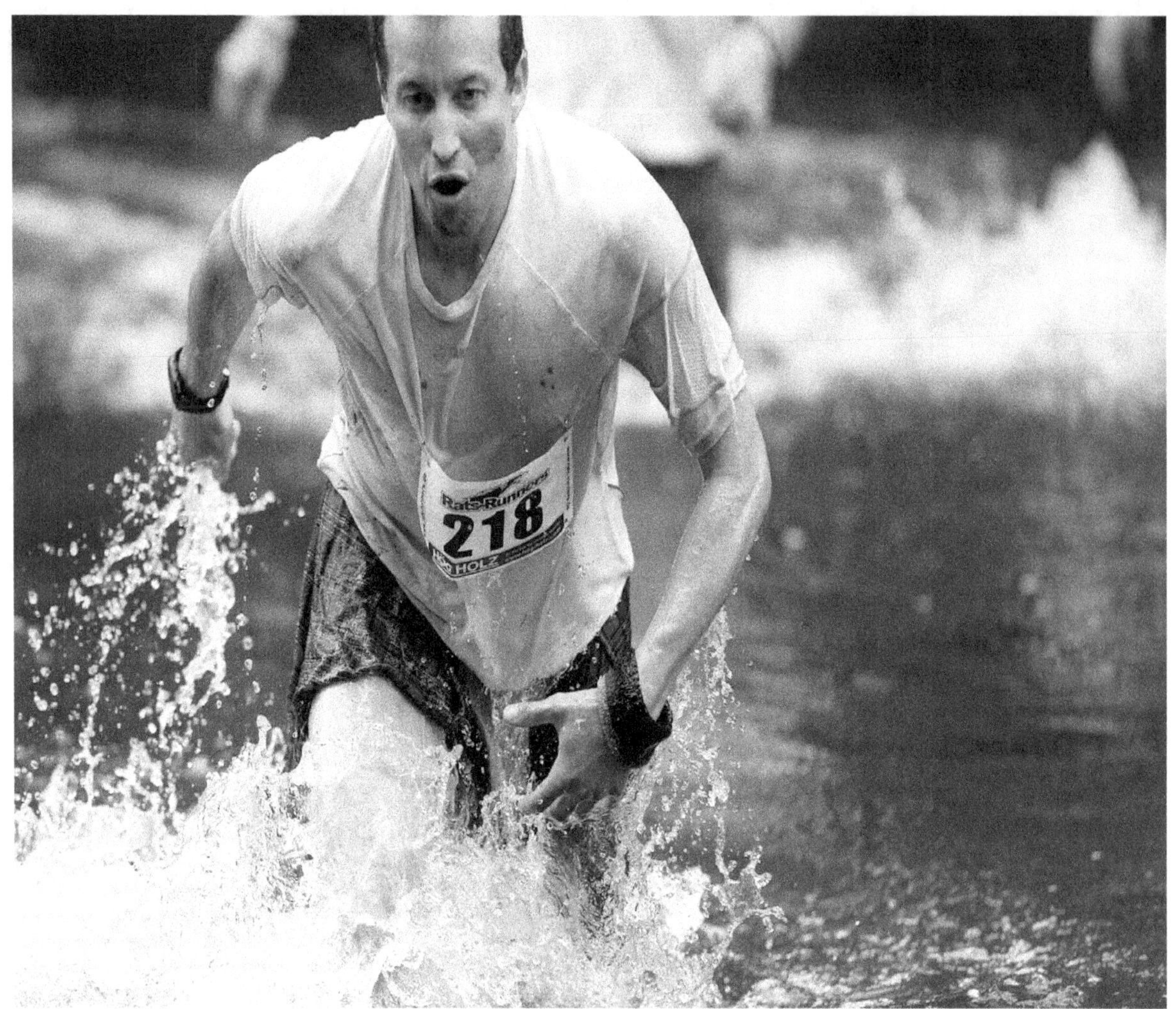

Building a positive mindset involves cultivating habits and attitudes that promote positivity. Tips for cultivating positivity include focusing on the present moment, practicing gratitude, and surrounding oneself with positive people. Self-compassion is also an important component of a positive mindset, as it involves treating oneself with kindness and understanding. Forgiveness and letting go of negative emotions can also help promote a positive mindset.

TIPS FOR CULTIVATING POSITIVITY

1. **Practice Gratitude**: Start each day by thinking about something that you are grateful for in your life. This could be anything from a warm cup of coffee to the people you love.

2. **Positive Self-Talk**: The way you talk to yourself has a big impact on your mood. Try to reframe negative thoughts into positive ones, and give yourself credit for your accomplishments.

3. **Find joy in the little things**: Take pleasure in the small moments that bring you joy. Whether it's a sunny day or a good meal, take time to appreciate the things that make you happy.

4. **Connect with others**: Reach out to friends or family members, or join a social group. Connecting with others can help to boost your mood and increase positivity.

5. **Take care of your body**: Exercise, eat healthy foods, and get enough sleep. When your body is healthy, your mind is more likely to be positive.

6. **Practice mindfulness**: Take time to focus on the present moment, without judgment. Mindfulness can help to reduce stress and increase positivity.

7. **Learn something new**: Challenge yourself to learn something new each day.

Whether it's a new skill or a new fact, learning can help to increase positivity and improve self-esteem.

8. **Find humor in situations**: Try to find the humor in everyday situations. Laughing can help to reduce stress and increase positivity.

9. **Set realistic goals**: Set goals that are achievable and work towards them. When you accomplish your goals, you will feel a sense of accomplishment and positivity.

10. **Take time for yourself**: Take time to do things that you enjoy, such as reading a book, taking a bath, or going for a walk. When you take care of yourself, you are more likely to feel positive and happy.

THE ROLE OF SELF-COMPASSION

1. **Reduces self-judgment**: Self-compassion helps us to be less critical of ourselves, reducing the self-judgment that can lead to negative self-talk and low self-esteem.

2. **Increases self-acceptance**: By accepting ourselves just as we are, flaws and all, we can begin to develop a healthier and more positive self-image.

3. **Promotes resilience**: Self-compassion helps us to bounce back from setbacks and challenges, building our resilience and helping us to persevere in the face of adversity.

4. **Cultivates empathy**: When we are kind and compassionate to ourselves, we are better able to extend that same empathy and compassion to others.

5. **Reduces stress and anxiety**: Self-compassion can help to reduce feelings of stress and anxiety by providing a calming and supportive presence within ourselves.

6. **Enhances self-care**: By treating ourselves with compassion and care, we are more likely to engage in healthy self-care practices, such as exercise, eating well, and getting enough rest.

7. **Supports personal growth**: Self-compassion helps us to let go of self-criticism and focus on growth and development, allowing us to reach our full potential.

8. **Promotes overall well-being**: By prioritizing self-compassion in our lives, we

can experience greater overall well-being, including increased happiness,

contentment, and satisfaction with life

9. **Provides emotional support**: Self-compassion allows us to provide ourselves

with the emotional support and kindness we need when we are struggling or

feeling down.

10. **Encourages self-awareness**: By practicing self-compassion, we can become

more aware of our thoughts, emotions, and behaviors, allowing us to make positive

changes in our lives.

PRACTICING FORGIVENESS AND LETTING GO

1. **Acknowledge and accept the pain**: Recognize the pain or hurt that has been caused and allow yourself to feel it fully.

2. **Focus on the present**: Reframe your thinking to focus on the present moment, rather than dwelling on the past.

3. **Practice self-compassion**: Treat yourself with kindness and compassion, recognizing that you are human and make mistakes.

4. **Let go of blame**: Release any blame or anger towards yourself or others, recognizing that everyone makes mistakes.

5. **Practice empathy**: Try to understand the perspective of the person who hurt you, even if you don't agree with their actions.

6. **Make amends if necessary**: If appropriate, make amends with the person who hurt you, whether it's through an apology or an act of kindness.

7. **Seek support**: Reach out to friends, family, or a therapist for support and guidance in the forgiveness process.

8. **Practice gratitude**: Focus on the positive aspects of your life and the things you are grateful for, rather than dwelling on the negative.

9. **Set healthy boundaries**: If necessary, set boundaries to protect yourself from further harm or hurt.

10. **Let go of resentment**: Release any resentment or grudges you may be holding

onto, recognizing that it only harms you in the long run.

CHAPTER 5

OVERCOMING OBSTACLES TO POSITIVE THINKING

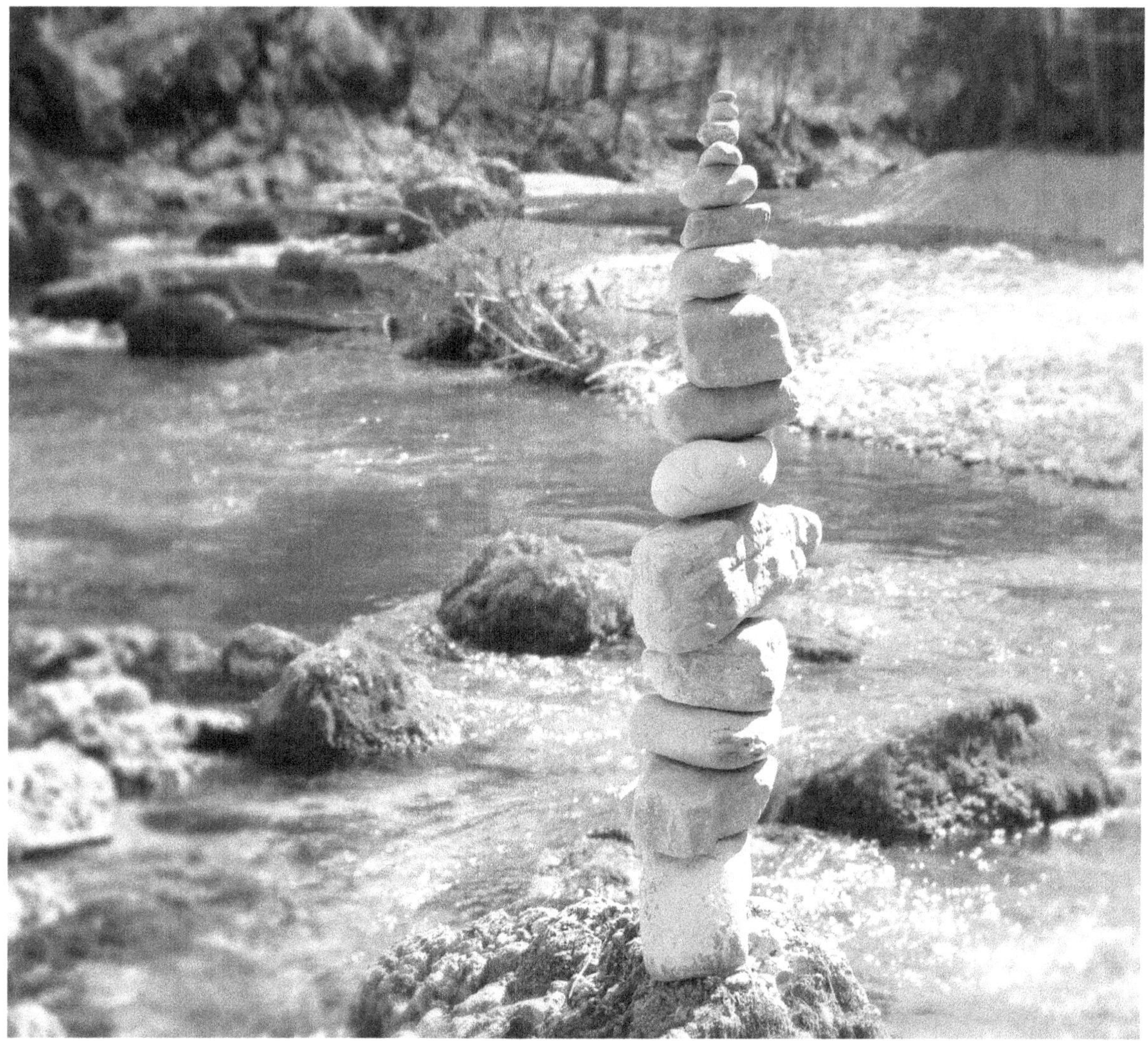

There are many obstacles that can interfere with positive thinking, including setbacks and failures, stress and anxiety, and negative beliefs and attitudes. Dealing with setbacks and failures involves reframing them as opportunities for growth and learning. Managing stress and anxiety can involve techniques such as mindfulness and meditation. Overcoming negative beliefs and attitudes can involve challenging them and replacing them with more positive ones.

DEALING WITH SETBACKS AND FAILURES

1. **Acknowledge and accept the setback**: Allow yourself to feel the disappointment or frustration that comes with failure, but don't dwell on it for too long.

2. **Reframe your mindset**: View setbacks as opportunities for growth and learning, rather than as a reflection of your worth or ability.

3. **Practice self-compassion**: Be kind and gentle with yourself, recognizing that failure is a normal part of the learning process.

4. **Seek support**: Reach out to friends, family, or a mentor for support and guidance in navigating the setback.

5. **Learn from the experience**: Identify what went wrong and what you can do differently next time to improve your chances of success.

6. **Stay focused on your goals**: Keep your eyes on the prize and remind yourself of what you're working towards.

7. **Stay positive**: Focus on the positive aspects of your life and the things you're grateful for, rather than dwelling on the negative.

8. **Take a break if needed**: If you're feeling overwhelmed or burnt out, take a

break to recharge and refresh your mindset.

9. **Keep moving forward**: Don't let setbacks hold you back or keep you from pursuing your goals. Keep pushing forward and taking action towards your goals.

10. **Embrace perseverance**: Success often requires persistence and perseverance in the face of setbacks and failures. Keep going and don't give up

MANAGING STRESS AND ANXIETY

1. **Practice deep breathing**: Take a few minutes to focus on your breath and take slow, deep breaths to calm your mind and body.

2. **Exercise regularly**: Regular physical activity can help to reduce stress and anxiety, as well as improve your overall physical health.

3. **Practice mindfulness**: Stay present in the moment and focus on the here and now, rather than worrying about the past or future.

4. **Get enough sleep**: Aim for 7-8 hours of sleep each night to help your body and mind recharge.

5. **Connect with others**: Spend time with loved ones, connect with friends, or join a support group to feel more connected and supported.

6. **Practice self-care**: Take time for yourself each day to engage in activities that bring you joy and relaxation, such as reading, taking a bath, or listening to music.

7. **Limit caffeine and alcohol**: Both caffeine and alcohol can increase feelings of anxiety and stress, so it's best to consume them in moderation or avoid them altogether.

8. **Stay organized**: Create a schedule or to-do list to help manage your time and reduce feelings of overwhelm.

9. **Seek professional help**: If you're struggling with anxiety or stress that is impacting your daily life, consider seeking professional help from a therapist or

mental health provider.

10. **Challenge negative thinking**: Practice reframing negative thoughts and focusing on positive aspects of a situation, rather than dwelling on the negative.

OVERCOMING NEGATIVE BELIEFS AND ATTITUDES

1. **Identify negative beliefs**: Start by identifying the negative beliefs or attitudes that are holding you back, such as "I'm not good enough" or "I always fail."

2. **Challenge those beliefs**: Question the validity of those negative beliefs and find evidence that contradicts them.

3. **Practice positive self-talk**: Replace negative self-talk with positive affirmations, such as "I am capable" or "I am deserving of success."

4. **Focus on strengths**: Instead of dwelling on weaknesses, focus on your strengths and positive qualities.

5. **Surround yourself with positivity**: Spend time with people who uplift and support you, and limit exposure to negative influences.

6. **Set achievable goals**: Break down larger goals into smaller, achievable steps to build confidence and momentum.

7. **Take action**: Take action towards your goals, even if it's just small steps, to build confidence and demonstrate to yourself that you are capable.

8. **Celebrate successes**: Celebrate even small successes and accomplishments, and use them to reinforce positive beliefs about yourself.

9. **Practice gratitude**: Focus on the positive aspects of your life and express gratitude for them regularly.

10. **Seek professional help**: If negative beliefs or attitudes are deeply ingrained and impacting your daily life, consider seeking professional help from a therapist or mental health provider

CHAPTER 6

MAINTAINING A POSITIVE OUTLOOK

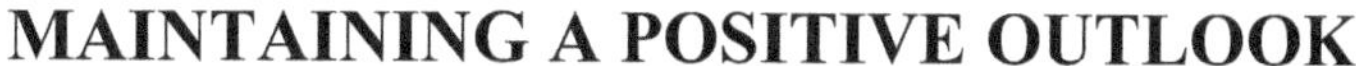

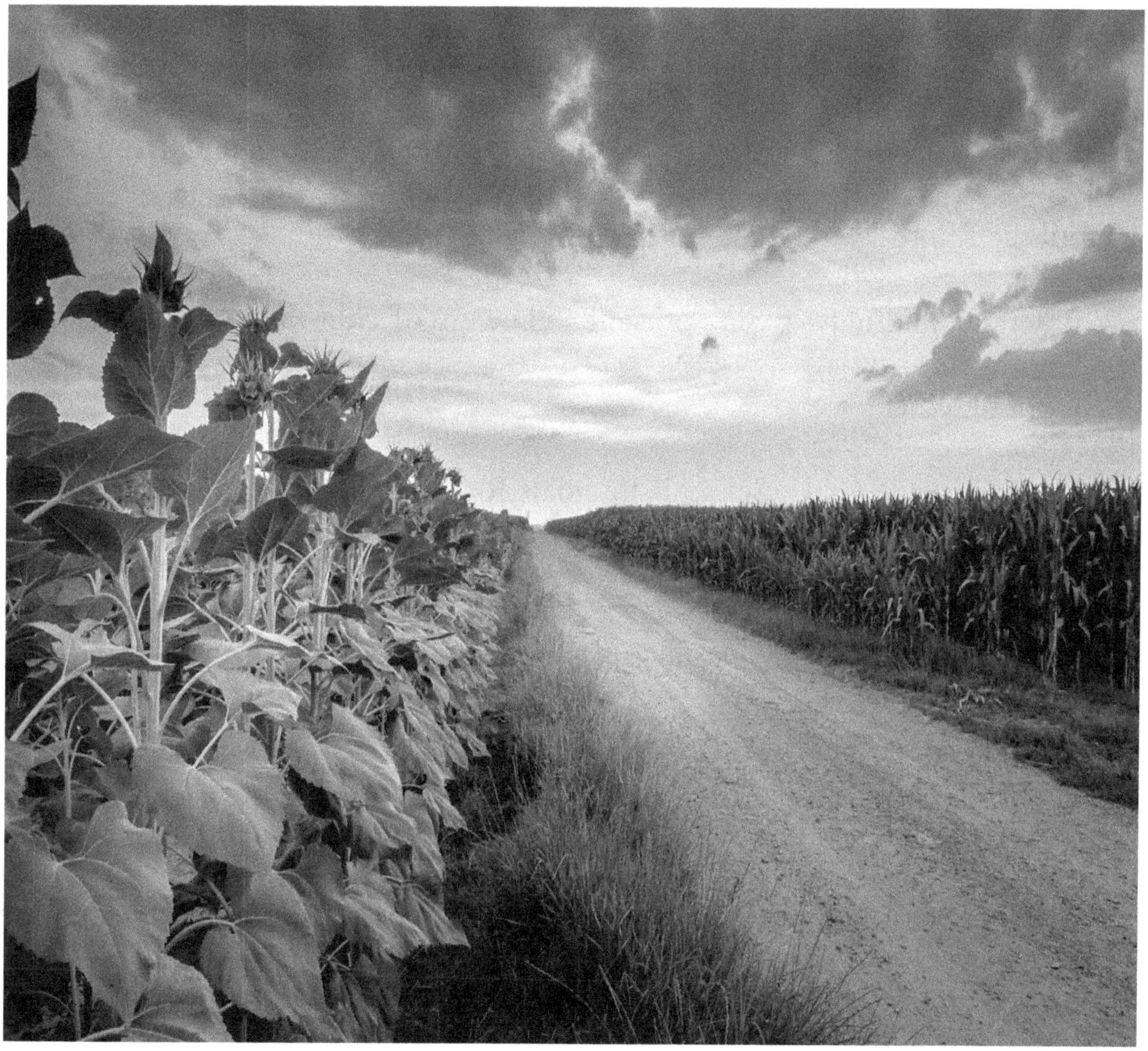

M aintaining a positive outlook over the long-term requires ongoing effort and commitment. Strategies for doing so include building resilience and coping skills, incorporating positive habits into daily life, and seeking support from others. Building resilience involves developing skills such as problem-solving, flexibility, and optimism. Coping skills can include techniques such as deep breathing, exercise, and spending time in nature.

STRATEGIES FOR STAYING POSITIVE OVER THE LONG-TERM

1. Focus on the present: Stay focused on the current moment and avoid worrying about the future.

2. Practice mindfulness: Stay present and aware of your thoughts and feelings without judgment.

3. Set achievable goals: Set realistic goals for the term and break them down into smaller, achievable steps.

4. Stay organized: Create a schedule or planner to help you stay on top of deadlines and assignments.

5. Take breaks: Take breaks throughout the day to recharge and avoid burnout.

6. Stay active: Regular exercise can help to reduce stress and anxiety, and improve your overall mood.

7. Connect with others: Stay connected with friends, family, or classmates for support and encouragement.

8. Practice self-care: Take care of yourself physically and mentally by getting enough sleep, eating well, and engaging in activities that bring you joy and relaxation.

9. Celebrate small victories: Recognize and celebrate even small achievements or

successes to stay motivated and positive.

10. Stay positive: Practice positive self-talk and focus on the positive aspects of your life, even in difficult times

BUILDING RESILIENCE AND COPING SKILLS

1. Cultivate a positive mindset: Focus on the positive aspects of situations and practice positive self-talk.

2. Practice mindfulness: Stay present in the moment and observe your thoughts and feelings without judgment.

3. Build a support system: Connect with friends, family, or a therapist for support and guidance during difficult times.

4. Set achievable goals: Set realistic goals and break them down into smaller, achievable steps.

5. Embrace challenges: See challenges as opportunities for growth and learning, rather than as obstacles.

6. Take care of yourself: Take care of your physical and mental health through regular exercise, healthy eating, and getting enough sleep.

7. Learn from mistakes: Use mistakes as opportunities to learn and grow, rather than dwelling on them.

8. Foster adaptability: Be open to change and willing to adapt to new situations.

9. Practice self-compassion: Be kind and gentle with yourself, recognizing that resilience is a process and that setbacks are a normal part of life.

10. Find meaning and purpose: Cultivate a sense of meaning and purpose in your life, and focus on what is important to you to help build resilience and cope with

adversity.

INCORPORATING POSITIVE HABITS INTO DAILY LIFE

1. **Start the day with positivity**: Begin each day with a positive affirmation or meditation to set a positive tone for the day ahead.

2. **Practice gratitude**: Take time each day to reflect on things you're grateful for, even small things.

3. **Set intentions**: Set daily intentions and goals to help stay focused and motivated throughout the day.

4. **Prioritize self-care**: Make time for self-care activities such as exercise, meditation, or a relaxing bath to improve overall well-being.

5. **Connect with others**: Connect with loved ones or friends to build positive relationships and social support.

6. **Build positive self-talk**: Replace negative self-talk with positive affirmations to boost self-esteem and confidence.

7. **Take breaks**: Take regular breaks throughout the day to rest and recharge, which can help reduce stress and increase productivity.

8. **Focus on the present**: Practice mindfulness and stay present in the moment, avoiding excessive worry or rumination.

9. **Limit negative influences**: Limit exposure to negative news, social media, or people who bring negativity into your life.

10. **Celebrate small wins**: Celebrate even small accomplishments and progress

towards goals, which can help build momentum and positivity

CHAPTER 7

BUILDING POSITIVE RELATIONSHIPS

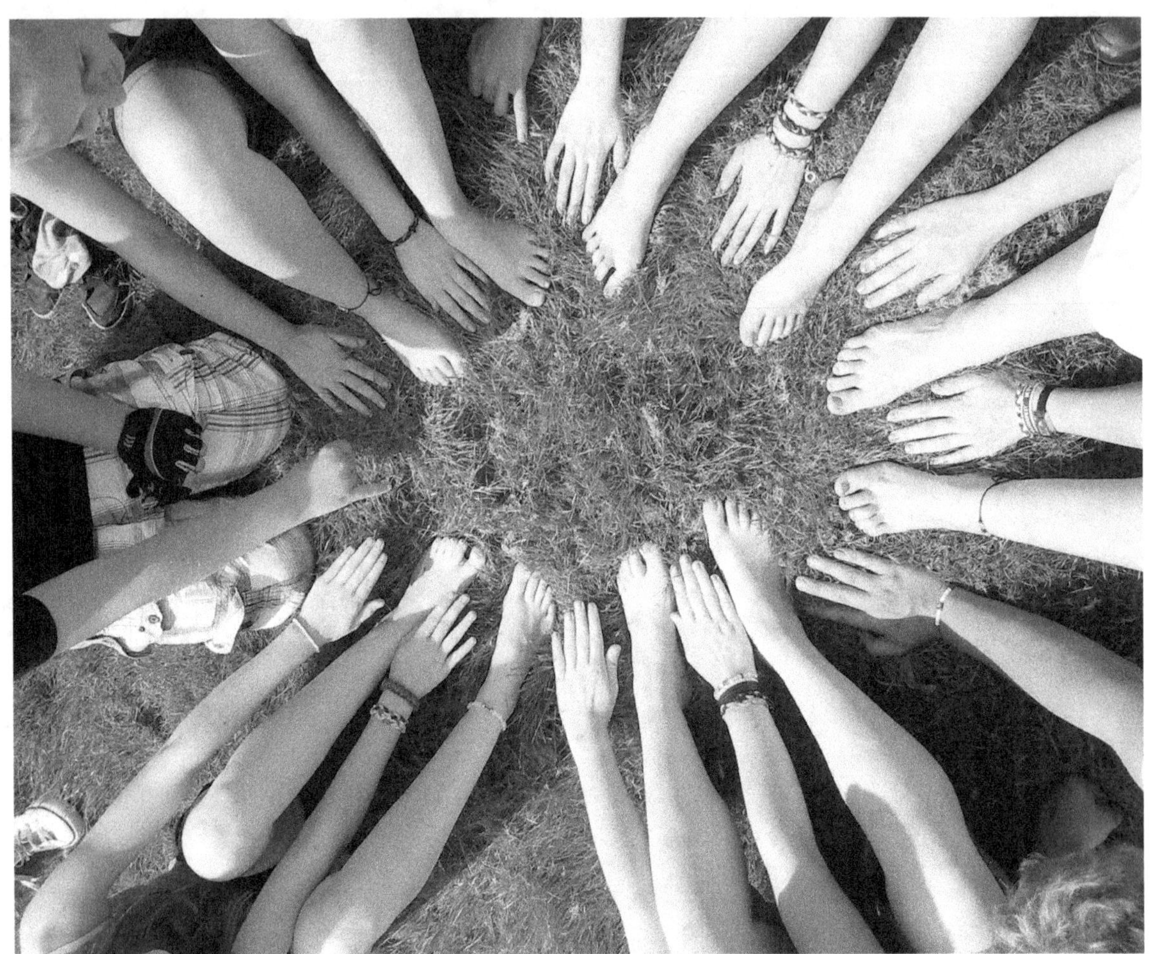

Positive relationships can have a significant impact on mental health, and it is important to cultivate and maintain them. Strategies for building positive relationships include being empathetic and kind, communicating effectively, and setting boundaries. Dealing with negative relationships may involve setting boundaries or seeking support from a therapist.

Practicing empathy and kindness towards others can help foster positive relationships and promote overall well-being

THE IMPACT OF POSITIVE RELATIONSHIPS ON MENTAL HEALTH

1. **Improved mood**: Positive relationships can have a positive impact on mood, leading to a decrease in symptoms of depression and anxiety.

2. **Increased self-esteem**: Being in positive relationships can improve feelings of self-worth and increase self-esteem.

3. **Reduced stress**: Positive relationships can provide emotional support during stressful times, leading to a reduction in stress levels.

4. **Enhanced coping skills**: Being in positive relationships can help individuals develop effective coping skills and increase resilience in the face of stressors.

5. **Better physical health**: Positive relationships have been linked to improved physical health, including a stronger immune system and a decreased risk of chronic illnesses.

6. **Improved communication skills**: Positive relationships can help individuals develop better communication skills, leading to more effective communication and reduced conflict.

7. **Increased social support**: Positive relationships can provide individuals with a sense of belonging and social support, which has been linked to better mental health outcomes.

8. **Greater happiness**: Positive relationships can bring joy and happiness to individuals, leading to an overall improvement in mental well-being.

9. **Improved self-care**: Positive relationships can encourage individuals to take better care of themselves, leading to improved mental and physical health outcomes.

10. **Greater resilience**: Positive relationships can help individuals build resilience and develop coping strategies, leading to better mental health outcomes in the face of adversity

STRATEGIES FOR BUILDING AND MAINTAINING POSITIVE RELATIONSHIPS

1. **Communication**: Effective communication is the foundation of any positive relationship. Listen actively, express yourself clearly, and work to understand the other person's perspective.

2. **Trust**: Building trust takes time, but it is crucial for maintaining positive relationships. Be reliable, keep your promises, and maintain confidentiality when appropriate.

3. **Respect**: Show respect for the other person's feelings, opinions, and boundaries. Avoid belittling or dismissing their views.

4. **Empathy**: Try to understand the other person's point of view and feelings. Show empathy by acknowledging their emotions and being supportive.

5. **Compromise**: Recognize that relationships require compromise and negotiation. Be open to finding solutions that work for both parties.

6. **Quality time**: Spending time together is important for building and maintaining positive relationships. Make time for meaningful conversations and shared activities.

7. **Appreciation**: Show appreciation for the other person and the things they do. Express gratitude for their contributions to the relationship.

8. **Forgiveness**: Forgiveness is essential for repairing relationships after conflicts.

Be willing to forgive and move forward, but also set boundaries to prevent the same mistakes from being repeated.

9. **Honesty**: Be honest and transparent in your communication. Avoid hiding your feelings or intentions.

10. **Commitment**: Building and maintaining positive relationships requires commitment. Show up consistently and invest time and effort in the relationship

DEALING WITH NEGATIVE RELATIONSHIPS AND SETTING BOUNDARIES

1. **Communicate your needs**: Be clear about your needs and expectations in the relationship. Communicate them assertively but respectfully.

2. **Set boundaries**: Once you've identified the problem and communicated your needs, set boundaries to protect yourself from negativity. This could involve limiting contact or reducing the amount of time spent with the person.

3. **Practice self-care**: It's important to take care of yourself when dealing with negative relationships. Prioritize self-care activities that help you relax and recharge.

4. **Seek support**: Reach out to friends or family members who can provide emotional support and help you stay accountable to your boundaries.

5. **Use "I" statements**: When communicating your needs and setting boundaries, use "I" statements to express how you feel rather than blaming the other person.

6. **Be consistent**: It's important to be consistent in your boundaries and communication. This helps the other person understand what to expect from you and what you expect from them.

7. **Be prepared for resistance**: Setting boundaries can sometimes be met with resistance or pushback from the other person. Be prepared to stand firm in your boundaries and assert your needs.

8. **Re-evaluate the relationship**: If the negativity continues despite setting boundaries, it may be time to re-evaluate the relationship and consider whether it's worth maintaining.

9. **Seek professional help**: If you're struggling to deal with negative relationships or set boundaries, consider seeking help from a therapist or counselor who can provide guidance and support

10. **Identify the problem**: Before setting boundaries, it's important to identify the problem in the relationship. Reflect on what's causing the negativity and how it's impacting you.

THE ROLE OF EMPATHY AND KINDNESS IN FOSTERING POSITIVE RELATIONSHIP

1. **Connection**: Kindness creates a connection between individuals that fosters a positive relationship. When people feel cared for and valued, they are more likely to maintain a positive relationship.

2. **Communication**: Empathy and kindness promote effective communication by creating a safe space where individuals can express themselves without fear of judgement.

3. **Trust**: When individuals show empathy and kindness towards one another, they build trust and strengthen their relationships.

4. **Resilience**: Empathy and kindness promote resilience in relationships by helping individuals navigate conflicts and challenges with understanding and compassion.

5. **Respect**: Empathy and kindness promote respect for others' perspectives, feelings, and boundaries. This fosters a positive relationship based on mutual respect and understanding.

6. **Support**: Kindness and empathy can provide emotional support during difficult times, leading to a stronger bond between individuals.

7. **Gratitude**: Kindness promotes gratitude, which can lead to a positive feedback loop in relationships. When individuals show kindness, they often receive kindness in return, leading to a stronger bond.

8. **Forgiveness**: Empathy and kindness can facilitate forgiveness by helping individuals understand the other person's perspective and experiences.

9. **Overall well-being**: Empathy and kindness can promote overall well-being by reducing stress and promoting positive emotions, leading to a healthier and happier relationship

10. **Understanding**: Empathy allows individuals to understand and relate to the feelings and experiences of others, leading to deeper connections and positive relationships.

CONCLUSION

THE IMPORTANCE OF POSITIVE THINKING FOR MENTAL HEALTH AND WELLBEING

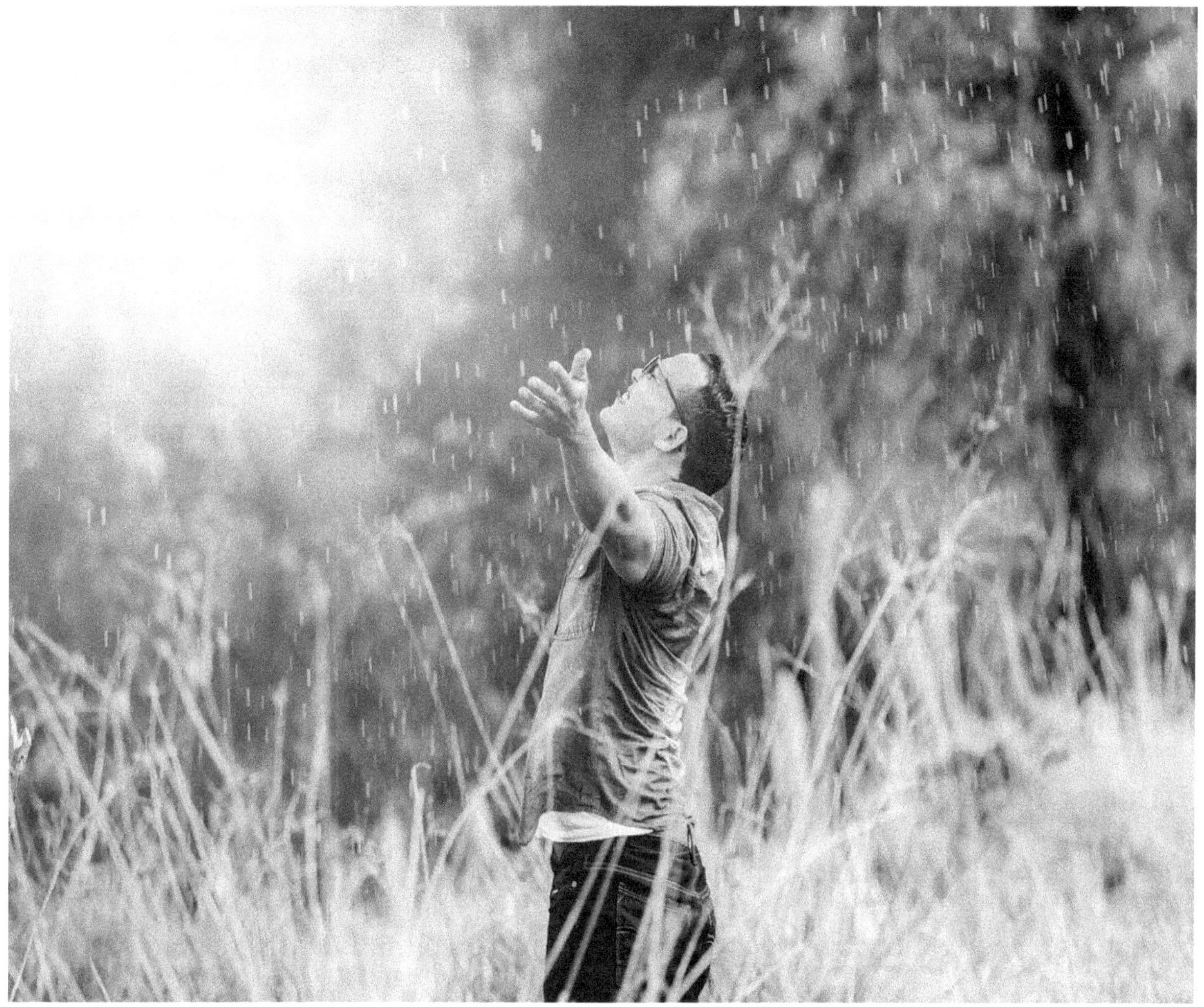

Positive thinking is an approach to life that emphasizes focusing on positive thoughts and experiences rather than dwelling on negative ones. It involves cultivating a mindset that looks for the good in situations and people, and finding opportunities for growth and learning in challenges.

Positive thinking has been linked to numerous benefits for mental health and well-being. Here are a few reasons why positive thinking is important:

1. **Reduces stress and anxiety**: Positive thinking can reduce stress and anxiety by helping individuals focus on the positive aspects of a situation. It can also help individuals reframe negative thoughts into more positive ones, reducing the impact of stress on mental health.

2. **Improves self-esteem**: Positive thinking can improve self-esteem by helping individuals focus on their strengths and accomplishments rather than their weaknesses and failures.

3. **Increases resilience**: Positive thinking can increase resilience by helping individuals develop a growth mindset that sees challenges as opportunities for growth and learning.

4. **Enhances relationships**: Positive thinking can enhance relationships by helping individuals approach others with compassion and understanding.

5. **Boosts mood**: Positive thinking can boost mood by promoting positive emotions such as happiness and contentment.

6. Increases motivation: Positive thinking can increase motivation by helping individuals focus on their goals and the steps they need to take to achieve them.

7. **Improves physical health**: Positive thinking has been linked to improved physical health outcomes such as lower blood pressure and reduced risk of cardiovascular disease.

Overall, positive thinking can have a significant impact on mental health and well-being. By cultivating a positive mindset, individuals can reduce stress, improve relationships, increase resilience, and enjoy a more fulfilling and satisfying life.

THE POWER OF SMALL STEPS TOWARDS POSITIVITY

The power of small steps towards positivity lies in the fact that these small actions, when practiced consistently over time, can lead to significant changes in our attitudes, behaviors, and overall well-being.

When we try to make big changes all at once, it can feel overwhelming and discouraging. We may find ourselves giving up quickly, feeling defeated, or feeling like the change is too difficult to sustain. By taking small steps, we can avoid these negative feelings and build momentum towards positive change.

Here are a few ways that small steps can lead to big changes:

1. **Building habits**: When we take small steps consistently over time, we can build new habits that become automatic and easy to maintain. For example, starting with a five-minute daily meditation practice can lead to a regular habit of mindfulness that improves our overall well-being.

2. **Breaking down big goals**: When we have a big goal in mind, it can be overwhelming to think about all the steps required to achieve it. By breaking it down into smaller, manageable steps, we can make progress towards the goal without feeling overwhelmed.

3. **Building confidence**: Achieving small goals can help us build confidence in ourselves and our abilities. This can lead to a positive cycle of taking on bigger challenges and achieving more over time.

4. **Increasing motivation**: Taking small steps towards positivity can increase our motivation by helping us see progress and feel a sense of accomplishment. This can inspire us to continue taking small steps and making positive changes in our lives.

Overall, the power of small steps towards positivity lies in the fact that they are easy to implement, sustainable, and can lead to significant improvements in our well-being over time. By focusing on small, manageable changes, we can build momentum towards positive change and enjoy a more fulfilling and satisfying life.

ENCOURAGEMENT TO CONTINUE PRACTISING POSITIVE THINKING

Practicing positive thinking can be challenging at times, but it's important to keep going because the benefits are truly worth it. Here are a few words of encouragement to help you continue practicing positive thinking:

1. **Remember the benefits**: When you're feeling discouraged, take a moment to remind yourself of the many benefits of positive thinking. These include reduced stress and anxiety, improved relationships, increased resilience, and more. Keep these benefits in mind as motivation to continue practicing.

2. **Celebrate small wins**: Don't overlook the small steps you take towards positive thinking. Celebrate each win, no matter how small, and use it as motivation to keep going.

3. **Be patient**: Positive thinking is a skill that takes time to develop. Be patient with yourself and remember that progress takes time.

4. **Stay mindful**: Mindfulness can help you stay present and focused on the positive aspects of your life. Practice mindfulness techniques such as deep breathing or meditation to help you stay centered and focused on the present moment.

5. **Surround yourself with positivity**: Surround yourself with people and things that bring positivity into your life. This can include supportive friends, inspiring books or podcasts, and uplifting music.

6. **Practice gratitude**: Gratitude is a powerful tool for promoting positive thinking. Take time each day to focus on the things you're grateful for, no matter how small they may seem.

7. **Keep a positive mindset**: When faced with challenges or setbacks, try to reframe them in a positive light. Look for opportunities for growth and learning in these situations and focus on the positive aspects of the experience.

Remember that practicing positive thinking is a journey, and it's okay to stumble along the way. Stay committed to your practice, celebrate small wins, and be patient with yourself. With time and effort, you can develop a more positive mindset and enjoy the many benefits that come with it.

Glossary

1. **Negative thoughts**: *Thoughts or mental patterns that create feelings of self-doubt, anxiety, depression, or other negative emotions.*

2. **Cognitive restructuring**: *A process of identifying and changing negative thought patterns and replacing them with more positive and realistic ones.*

3. **Mindfulness**: *A practice of staying present in the moment and being aware of one's thoughts and emotions without judgment.*

4. **Acceptance**: *A practice of acknowledging and accepting one's thoughts and emotions, rather than resisting or avoiding them.*

5. **Reframing**: *A technique of changing the perspective on a situation or thought to see it in a more positive or constructive light.*

6. **Gratitude**: *A practice of focusing on the positive aspects of one's life and feeling grateful for them.*

7. **Self-compassion**: *A practice of treating oneself with kindness and understanding, rather than self-criticism or judgment.*

8. **Relaxation techniques**: *Practices such as meditation, deep breathing, or progressive muscle relaxation that promote relaxation and reduce stress and anxiety.*

9. **Positive self-talk**: *The practice of using positive affirmations and statements to counter negative self-talk and build self-esteem.*

10. **Behavioral activation**: *A technique of engaging in positive activities and behaviors to improve mood and reduce negative thoughts and emotions.*

11. **Resilience**: *The ability to bounce back from setbacks or challenges and*

maintain a positive outlook.

12. Emotional regulation: The ability to identify and manage one's emotions in a healthy and constructive way.

13. **Coping skills**: Techniques and strategies for managing stress, anxiety, and other negative emotions.

14. **Self-care**: Activities and practices that promote physical, emotional, and mental well-being, such as exercise, healthy eating, and rest.

15. **Mind-body connection**: The link between physical health and mental and emotional well-being, and the impact that one has on the other.

16. **Support network**: The people in one's life who provide emotional support, encouragement, and guidance during difficult times.

17. **Positive psychology**: The scientific study of the factors that contribute to well-being and happiness, and the techniques and strategies for cultivating a positive mindset.

18. **Therapy**: A professional intervention that provides support and guidance for managing mental health issues and improving emotional well-being.

19. **Journaling**: A practice of writing down thoughts, emotions, and experiences as a means of processing and reflecting on them.

20. **Gratitude journaling**: A practice of writing down things for which one is grateful, as a way of focusing on the positive aspects of life and promoting well-being.

21. **Mindset**: The set of beliefs and attitudes that shape how one approaches and

responds to situations and challenges.

*22. **Goal-setting**: The process of identifying specific, measurable, achievable, relevant, and time-bound goals, and developing a plan to achieve them.*

*23. **Positive affirmations**: Positive statements or phrases that are repeated to oneself in order to promote a positive mindset and belief in oneself.*

*24. **Resourcing**: The practice of identifying and utilizing personal strengths and resources, such as skills, abilities, and social support, to overcome challenges and achieve goals.*

*25. **Compassion-focused therapy**: A therapeutic approach that emphasizes the importance of self-compassion and empathy in overcoming negative thoughts and emotions.*

*26. **Cognitive-behavioral therapy (CBT):** A therapeutic approach that focuses on identifying and changing negative thought patterns and behaviors in order to improve mental health and emotional well-being.*

*27. **Mindfulness-based cognitive therapy (MBCT):** A therapeutic approach that combines mindfulness practices with cognitive-behavioral techniques to help individuals manage negative thoughts and emotions.*

*28. **Graded exposure therapy**: A therapeutic approach that gradually exposes individuals to anxiety-provoking situations or stimuli, in order to reduce fear and anxiety.*

*29. **Positive reframing**: A technique of identifying positive aspects or opportunities in a negative situation or thought, in order to shift perspective and promote a more positive mindset.*

30. ***Self-awareness***: *The ability to recognize and understand one's own thoughts, emotions, and behaviors, and their impact on oneself and others.*

31. ***Self-talk***: *The internal dialogue that occurs within an individual's mind, which can be either positive or negative.*

32. ***Cognitive distortions***: *Unhelpful or inaccurate thought patterns that can contribute to negative emotions and behavior, such as all-or-nothing thinking, catastrophizing, or personalization.*

33. ***Positive reappraisal***: *A technique of reframing a negative situation by focusing on positive aspects or potential outcomes.*

34. ***Assertiveness***: *The ability to express one's needs, opinions, and boundaries in a clear and respectful manner, while also considering the needs of others.*

35. ***Active listening***: *A communication technique that involves fully focusing on and understanding another person's message, without judgment or interruption.*

36. ***Mind-wandering***: *The tendency for one's thoughts to drift away from the present moment, which can contribute to negative emotions and distract from important tasks.*

37. ***Attentional bias***: *The tendency for one's attention to be drawn towards negative or threatening stimuli, which can contribute to anxiety and other negative emotions.*

38. ***Rumination***: *The tendency to excessively dwell on negative thoughts or*

experiences, which can contribute to depression and other negative emotions.

*39. **Self-reflection**: The practice of examining one's own thoughts, emotions, and behaviors in order to gain insight and promote personal growth.*

*40. **Emotional intelligence**: The ability to recognize, understand, and manage one's own emotions, as well as the emotions of others, in order to improve interpersonal relationships and communication*

*41. **Cognitive restructuring**: A therapeutic technique that involves identifying and challenging negative thought patterns, and replacing them with more positive and accurate ones.*

*42. **Mind-body practices**: Techniques that involve the use of physical and mental exercises to promote relaxation, reduce stress, and improve mental and emotional well-being, such as yoga, tai chi, or meditation.*

*43. **Emotional support animals**: Animals, such as dogs or cats, that are trained to provide comfort, companionship, and emotional support to individuals with mental health conditions.*

*44. **Social comparison**: The tendency to evaluate one's own abilities, achievements, and circumstances in comparison to others, which can contribute to negative emotions and self-doubt.*

*45. **Graded exposure therapy**: A therapeutic approach that gradually exposes individuals to anxiety-provoking situations or stimuli, in order to reduce fear and anxiety.*

*46. **Cognitive fusion**: The tendency to become overly identified with one's thoughts* *and emotions, which can contribute to negative self-talk and self-doubt.*

*47. **Acceptance and Commitment Therapy (ACT):** A therapeutic approach that focuses on developing mindfulness and acceptance skills, and committing to actions that align with one's values, in order to overcome negative thoughts and emotions.*

*48. **Positive visualization**: A technique of imagining positive outcomes or scenarios, in order to promote a positive mindset and increase motivation.*

*49. **Proactive coping**: The practice of anticipating and preparing for future stressors or challenges, in order to reduce the impact of negative emotions and improve resilience.*

*50. **Behavioral activation**: A therapeutic approach that focuses on identifying and engaging in pleasurable and meaningful activities, in order to improve mood and reduce negative emotions.*

SUMMARY

"Positive Thinking" is the latest book by Sagittarius Partey, a renowned self-help author and motivational speaker. In this inspiring work, he shares their personal journey of overcoming adversity and the power of positive thinking in achieving success.

The book begins with an introduction to the concept of positive thinking and its many benefits, including increased happiness, better health, and greater success. He then delves into their own experiences with negative thinking and how it held them back in life. They share stories of how they overcame these negative thoughts and replaced them with positive ones, leading to a more fulfilling life.

Throughout the book, he provides practical tips and techniques for cultivating a positive mindset, such as gratitude journaling, affirmations, and visualization. They also share insights from experts in the fields of psychology and neuroscience, to explain the science behind positive thinking and how it can literally rewire the brain for greater happiness and success.

One of the standout features of "Positive Thinking" is he's engaging writing style and relatable anecdotes. They use real-life examples and stories to illustrate their points, making the book both informative and entertaining to read.

Whether you are struggling with negative thoughts and emotions or simply looking for ways to improve your life, "Positive Thinking" is a must-read. With its inspiring message and practical advice, this book will help you transform your mindset and achieve your goals.

AUTHOR

"Positive Thinking" is an uplifting and inspiring book that offers practical advice and insights on how to cultivate a positive mindset. **Sagittarius Partey** draws on their own experiences and expertise to provide readers with a valuable resource for overcoming negative thoughts and achieving success. Their writing is engaging and relatable, making the book accessible to readers of all backgrounds and ages.

I highly recommend "Positive Thinking" to anyone who wants to live a happier, more fulfilling life – **Java Color**

This book will help you unlock your potential and unleash the power of positive thinking – **May Johnson**